The Art of Emotional Mastery:

A Guide to Harnessing Your Feelings and Transforming Your Life

By

Luke L. Perry

Contents

Introduction:

Welcome to "The Art of Emotional Mastery: Strategies for Understanding and Managing Your Feelings." Emotions are an integral part of our lives, shaping our thoughts, actions, and relationships. They can be a source of great joy, but they can also be a source of pain and distress.

Emotions are not always easy to manage, and many of us struggle to understand and express them. We may feel overwhelmed by our emotions, and they may dictate our behavior in ways that we do not understand or cannot control. However, mastering our emotions is crucial to our overall well-being and success in life.

This book is designed to help you understand and manage your emotions effectively. We will explore the nature of emotions, how they arise, and their impact on our lives. We will also discuss various strategies and techniques that can help you develop emotional intelligence, cultivate positive emotions, and overcome negative ones.

Throughout the book, you will learn how to recognize and understand your emotions, identify triggers that cause them, and develop strategies to manage them effectively. You will also discover practical techniques for dealing with difficult emotions like anger, fear, and anxiety.

By the end of this book, you will have a deeper

understanding of your emotions and the tools to manage them effectively. Whether you're seeking greater emotional resilience, better relationships, or simply a happier and more fulfilling life, "The Art of Emotional Mastery" is the guide you need.

PART ONE: Understanding Emotions

Chapter 1:
What Are Emotions?

Emotions are complex psychological and physiological responses to stimuli in the environment, such as events, experiences, or thoughts. They involve a wide range of subjective feelings, including joy, love, anger, fear, sadness, and disgust, among others.

Emotions are not just limited to feelings, they also involve physical and behavioral responses that accompany those feelings. For example, when we experience fear, we may feel our heart race, our palms sweat, and our body tense up. We may also have a strong urge to flee from the source of our fear.

Emotions can be triggered by external events or internal thoughts and beliefs, and they can vary in intensity and duration. They are also influenced by individual factors such as personality, culture, and personal history.

Emotions serve a purpose in our lives, helping us to navigate and respond to the world around us. They can motivate us to take action, communicate our needs and desires, and help us form relationships with others. However, emotions can also be challenging to manage and regulate, and they can sometimes lead to negative consequences if not handled effectively.

Chapter 2:
The Role of Emotions in Our Lives

Emotions play a significant role in our lives, influencing our thoughts, behaviors, and overall well-being. In this chapter, we will explore the various ways emotions impact us and why they are essential for our daily functioning.

Communicating our needs and desires

One of the primary functions of emotions is to communicate our needs and desires to others. For example, when we feel hungry, we may experience the emotion of hunger, which signals to us that we need to eat. Hunger also communicates our needs to others, who may respond by offering us food or helping us find a way to satisfy our hunger.

Guiding our decision-making

Emotions can also guide our decision-making by influencing our preferences and choices. For example, if we feel happy when spending time with friends, we may choose to prioritize social activities over other obligations. Conversely, if we feel anxious about a particular task, we may avoid it or seek out help to manage our anxiety.

Motivating us to take action

Emotions can also motivate us to take action in response to a particular situation. For example, if we feel afraid, we may take steps to protect ourselves or seek out safety. Similarly, if we feel excited about a new opportunity, we may be more likely to pursue it with enthusiasm.

Providing us with valuable feedback

Emotions can also provide us with valuable feedback about our experiences and relationships. For example, if we feel happy and fulfilled in a particular job, it may be a sign that we are on the right career path. Alternatively, if we feel unhappy and unfulfilled in a relationship, it may be a sign that it is time to make a change.

In summary, emotions serve a crucial role in our lives, helping us communicate our needs, guide our decision-making, motivate us to take action, and provide us with valuable feedback about our experiences and relationships. While emotions can sometimes be challenging to manage, developing emotional intelligence and learning effective emotional regulation strategies can help us reap the benefits of our emotions and live happier, more fulfilling lives.

Chapter 3:
How Emotions Are Generated

In this chapter, we will explore how emotions are generated and the various factors that contribute to their formation.

Appraisal Theory

Appraisal theory proposes that emotions are generated through a cognitive evaluation of a particular event or situation. In other words, the way we interpret and evaluate a situation determines the emotions we experience. For example, if we interpret a situation as threatening, we may experience fear, while if we interpret it as rewarding, we may experience happiness.

Social Constructivism

Social constructivism suggests that emotions are socially constructed, meaning they are influenced by cultural and social factors. Different cultures may have different emotional expressions, and the way we learn to express and understand emotions is shaped by our social interactions and cultural background.

Evolutionary Theory

Evolutionary theory suggests that emotions have evolved over time to help us adapt to our environment and survive. For example, fear may have evolved as a response to potential threats, while joy may have evolved as a way to reinforce positive behaviors and experiences.

Neuroscience

Neuroscience research has shown that emotions are generated by the interplay between various brain structures and neurotransmitters. The amygdala, for example, is a key brain structure involved in processing emotions, particularly fear. Neurotransmitters like dopamine and serotonin also play a crucial role in regulating our emotions.

Personal Experience

Finally, personal experience plays a crucial role in generating emotions. Our past experiences and memories can influence the way we interpret and respond to new situations, and can even shape our emotional responses over time.

In summary, emotions are generated through a complex interplay of cognitive, social, evolutionary, and neurobiological factors, as well as personal experience. Understanding the factors that contribute to emotional generation can help us better understand our own emotions and develop effective emotional

regulation strategies.

Chapter 4:
The Science of Emotions

In this chapter, we will delve deeper into the science of emotions, exploring the biological and psychological processes that underlie our emotional experiences.

The Amygdala

The amygdala is a key brain structure involved in processing emotions, particularly fear. It is part of the limbic system and plays a crucial role in determining whether a situation is potentially threatening or rewarding. The amygdala also plays a role in our emotional memories and helps us form associations between emotions and experiences.

Neurotransmitters

Neurotransmitters are chemical messengers that transmit signals between neurons in the brain. Several neurotransmitters are involved in regulating our emotions, including serotonin, dopamine, and norepinephrine. Imbalances in these neurotransmitters can contribute to mood disorders such as depression and anxiety.

The Autonomic Nervous System

The autonomic nervous system is responsible for regulating many of our bodily functions, including our emotional responses. It is divided into two branches: the sympathetic nervous system, which prepares the body for action during stress or danger (the fight or flight response), and the parasympathetic nervous system, which helps us relax and recover after stress. These two systems work together to regulate our emotional responses and physiological reactions.

Emotional Regulation

Emotional regulation refers to the processes by which we manage and modify our emotional experiences. Strategies for emotional regulation can include cognitive reappraisal (changing the way we think about a situation), behavioral changes (engaging in activities that promote positive emotions), and mindfulness practices (cultivating present-moment awareness and non-judgmental acceptance of our emotions).

The Social Nature of Emotions

Emotions are inherently social and are shaped by our interactions with others. Social factors such as culture, social norms, and interpersonal relationships can all influence the way we express and understand emotions. For example, cultural differences in emotional expression can lead to misunderstandings and miscommunication between individuals from different cultures.

In summary, the science of emotions is a complex and multidisciplinary field that encompasses various biological, psychological, and social factors. Understanding these factors can help us better understand our emotional experiences and develop effective emotional regulation strategies.

Part 2: Developing Emotional Intelligence

Chapter 5:
What Is Emotional Intelligence?

In this chapter, we will explore the concept of emotional intelligence, including its definition, components, and importance for personal and professional success.

Definition of Emotional Intelligence

Emotional intelligence (EI) refers to the ability to perceive, understand, and manage one's own emotions, as well as the emotions of others. It involves a range of skills, including emotional awareness, empathy, self-regulation, and social skills.

Components of Emotional Intelligence

There are several models of emotional intelligence, but most include the following components:

Self-awareness: the ability to recognize and understand one's own emotions and how they impact behavior and decision-making.

Self-regulation: the ability to manage one's own emotions and impulses, and to adapt to changing circumstances.

Motivation: the drive to achieve goals and persist in the face of challenges.

Empathy: the ability to understand and relate to the emotions of others.

Social skills: the ability to communicate effectively, build and maintain relationships, and work collaboratively with others.

Importance of Emotional Intelligence

Research has shown that emotional intelligence is a strong predictor of personal and professional success. Individuals with high EI are more likely to be effective leaders, have better relationships, and be more resilient in the face of stress and adversity. Additionally, organizations with emotionally intelligent leaders and employees tend to have better morale, productivity, and overall performance.

Developing Emotional Intelligence

While some aspects of emotional intelligence may be innate, it is also a skill that can be developed and improved through practice and training. Strategies for developing emotional intelligence can include mindfulness practices, empathy training, and communication and conflict resolution skills.

In summary, emotional intelligence is a key factor in personal and professional success and involves a range of skills related to emotional awareness, self-regulation, empathy, and social skills. Developing emotional intelligence can lead to better relationships, increased resilience, and improved performance in both personal and professional settings.

Chapter 6:
The Five Components of Emotional Intelligence

In this chapter, we will be looking at the five components of emotional intelligence and exploring strategies for developing each component.

Self-Awareness

Self-awareness is the ability to recognize and understand one's own emotions and their impact on behavior and decision-making. Strategies for developing self-awareness can include:

Mindfulness practices, such as meditation or journaling to increase awareness of thoughts and emotions.

Reflection and self-assessment exercises,

such as asking for feedback from others or identifying personal strengths and weaknesses.

Keeping a mood diary or tracking emotions

throughout the day to increase awareness of emotional patterns.

Self-Regulation

Self-regulation is the ability to manage one's own

emotions and impulses and to adapt to changing circumstances. Strategies for developing self-regulation can include:

Deep breathing or other relaxation techniques to reduce stress and increase emotional control.

Cognitive reappraisal, or changing the way we think about a situation to reduce negative emotions and promote positive ones.

Developing healthy habits, such as exercise and sleep, to improve emotional regulation and reduce stress.

Motivation

Motivation refers to the drive to achieve goals and persist in the face of challenges. Strategies for developing motivation can include:

Setting clear, achievable goals and tracking progress toward them.

Cultivating a growth mindset, or the belief that one's abilities can be developed through effort and learning.

Focusing on intrinsic motivation, or the internal drive to do something for its own sake, rather than relying solely on external rewards.

Empathy

Empathy is the ability to understand and relate to the emotions of others. Strategies for developing empathy can include:

Active listening and non-judgmental communication to better understand others' perspectives.

Practicing perspective- taking, or imagining oneself in another's situation, to increase empathy and understanding.

Engaging in community service or volunteering to increase exposure to diverse perspectives and experiences.

Social Skills

Social skills refer to the ability to communicate effectively, build and maintain relationships, and work collaboratively with others. Strategies for developing social skills can include:

Practicing effective communication, such as active listening, assertiveness, and conflict resolution.

Building and maintaining relationships through networking, mentoring, and social support.

Developing leadership skills, such as delegation,

decision-making, and team building.

In summary, the five components of emotional intelligence - self-awareness, self-regulation, motivation, empathy, and social skills - are critical skills for personal and professional success. Developing these skills can lead to better relationships, increased resilience, and improved performance in various areas of life.

Chapter 7:
Self-Awareness:
Recognizing Your Emotions

In this chapter, we will focus on the first component of emotional intelligence - self-awareness - and explore strategies for recognizing and understanding our own emotions.

The Importance of Self-Awareness

Self-awareness is a foundational component of emotional intelligence. It allows us to recognize our own emotions and how they influence our behavior, thoughts, and decisions. Without self-awareness, we may act impulsively or unconsciously, and struggle to manage our emotions effectively.

Recognizing Your Emotions

Recognizing your emotions involves paying attention to your feelings and bodily sensations, and identifying the specific emotions you are experiencing. Some strategies for recognizing your emotions can include:

Mindfulness practices, such as meditation or deep breathing, to increase present-moment awareness of bodily sensations and emotions.

Labeling emotions using a feelings wheel or other resource to increase awareness of specific emotions and their nuances.

Seeking feedback from others, such as asking a trusted friend or family member to provide honest observations of your emotional patterns.

Understanding Your Emotions

Once you have recognized your emotions, the next step is to understand them. This involves exploring the root causes of your emotions and how they may be related to your thoughts, beliefs, and past experiences. Strategies for understanding your emotions can include:

Journaling or reflective writing to explore the

origins and impact of your emotions.

Working with a therapist or counselor to gain deeper insight into emotional patterns and develop coping strategies. **Engaging in self-reflection exercises**, such as asking yourself why you feel a certain way or identifying the triggers for your emotions.

Managing Your Emotions

Self-awareness is also critical for managing your emotions effectively. By recognizing and understanding your emotions, you can develop strategies for regulating them and responding to them in healthy ways. Strategies for managing your emotions can include:

Developing coping strategies, such as deep breathing, exercise, or visualization techniques, to reduce the intensity of negative emotions.

Practicing cognitive reappraisal, or changing the way you think about a situation, to reduce negative emotions and promote positive ones.

Engaging in self-care activities, such as spending time in nature or engaging in creative pursuits, to boost positive emotions and reduce stress.

In summary, self-awareness is a critical component of emotional intelligence that involves recognizing and understanding your own emotions. Strategies for recognizing and understanding your emotions can include mindfulness practices, seeking feedback, and engaging in self-reflection exercises. By developing self-awareness, you can better manage your emotions and improve your overall well-being.

Chapter 8:
Self-Regulation: Managing Your Emotions

In this chapter, we will focus on the second component of emotional intelligence - self-regulation - and explore strategies for managing our emotions in healthy and effective ways.

The Importance of Self-Regulation

Self-regulation is the ability to manage and regulate

one's own emotions, thoughts, and behaviors. It involves being able to control impulsive reactions, manage stress and anxiety, and maintain a positive outlook. Developing self-regulation skills can help you improve your relationships, achieve your goals, and enhance your overall well-being.

Strategies for Self-Regulation

There are several strategies you can use to develop self-regulation skills, including:

Mindfulness meditation: Mindfulness meditation involves focusing your attention on the present moment, observing your thoughts and emotions without judgment, and cultivating a sense of calm and relaxation. Regular practice can help you regulate your emotions, reduce stress, and improve your overall well-being.

Emotional reappraisal: Emotional reappraisal involves reinterpreting or reframing a situation in a more positive light, which can help you regulate negative emotions and reduce stress. For example, if you receive negative feedback at work, you can try to view it as an opportunity for growth and learning.

Cognitive restructuring:

Cognitive restructuring involves identifying and challenging negative thought patterns and replacing them with more positive and realistic ones. This can help you regulate your emotions and improve your overall well-being.

Physical activity: Engaging in regular physical activity, such as exercise or yoga, can help you regulate your emotions, reduce stress, and improve your overall well-being.

The Role of Self-Care in Self-Regulation

Self-care is an important aspect of self-regulation. Taking care of your physical, emotional, and mental health can help you better manage your emotions and reduce stress. Some self-care strategies you can use to support self-regulation include:

Getting enough sleep: Getting enough restful sleep can help you regulate your emotions, reduce stress, and improve your overall well-being.

Eating a healthy diet: Eating a balanced and nutritious diet can help you regulate your emotions, reduce stress, and improve your overall well-being.

Engaging in leisure activities: Engaging in hobbies and leisure activities that bring you joy and relaxation can help you reduce stress and improve your overall well-being.

In summary, self-regulation is a critical component of emotional intelligence that involves managing and regulating one's own emotions, thoughts, and behaviors. Strategies for self-regulation can include mindfulness meditation, emotional reappraisal, cognitive restructuring, and physical activity. Practicing self-care is also important for supporting self-regulation and improving overall well-being.

Chapter 9:
Motivation: Channeling Your Emotions

In this chapter, we will explore the third component of emotional intelligence - motivation - and how to channel our emotions to drive us toward our goals.

The Importance of Motivation

Motivation is the driving force behind our behaviors, thoughts, and emotions. It is what propels us toward our goals and keeps us moving forward. Developing motivation skills can help us achieve our goals, improve our relationships, and enhance our overall well-being.

Strategies for Motivation

There are several strategies you can use to develop motivation skills, including:

Setting SMART goals: Setting specific, measurable, achievable, relevant, and time-bound (SMART) goals can help you stay motivated and focused on achieving your objectives.

Creating a positive mindset: Cultivating a positive mindset can help you stay motivated and overcome obstacles. This involves focusing on your strengths, having a growth mindset, and reframing negative thoughts into positive ones.

Using visualization techniques: Visualizing yourself achieving your goals can help you stay motivated and focused on your objectives.

Seeking support: Surrounding yourself with

positive and supportive people can help you stay motivated and overcome obstacles.

The Role of Emotions in Motivation

Emotions play a crucial role in motivation. They can either drive us toward our goals or hinder our progress. Understanding our emotions and how to regulate them can help us use them as a tool to fuel our motivation.

The Importance of Self-Compassion in Motivation

Self-compassion is an important aspect of motivation. It involves treating ourselves with kindness, empathy, and understanding. Practicing self-compassion can help us overcome obstacles, bounce back from failure, and stay motivated toward our goals.

In summary, motivation is a critical component of emotional intelligence that involves channeling our emotions toward achieving our goals. Strategies for motivation can include setting SMART goals, cultivating a positive mindset, using visualization techniques, and seeking support. Understanding the role of emotions and practicing self-compassion are also important for enhancing motivation skills and achieving our objectives.

Chapter 10:
Empathy: Understanding Others' Emotions

In this chapter, we will explore the fourth component of emotional intelligence - empathy - and how to develop our ability to understand and connect with others' emotions.

The Importance of Empathy

Empathy is the ability to understand and connect with others' emotions. It is a crucial component of healthy relationships and effective communication. Developing empathy skills can help us build stronger connections with others, improve our social interactions, and enhance our overall well-being.

Types of Empathy

There are three types of empathy: cognitive empathy, emotional empathy, and compassionate empathy.

Cognitive empathy involves understanding others' emotions from a logical perspective.

Emotional empathy involves feeling others' emotions as if they were our own.

Compassionate empathy involves feeling others' emotions and taking action to help alleviate their suffering.

Strategies for Developing Empathy

There are several strategies you can use to develop empathy skills, including:

Listening actively: Listening actively to others' perspectives and experiences can help you understand their emotions and connect with them on a deeper level.

Practicing perspective-taking: Imagining yourself

in others' shoes can help you understand their emotions and experiences.

Showing compassion: Showing compassion towards others' suffering can help you connect with their emotions and provide support.

Cultivating self-awareness: Understanding and regulating your own emotions can help you empathize with others and connect with them on a deeper level.

The Benefits of Empathy

Developing empathy skills can have numerous benefits, including:

Improved relationships: Empathy can help us understand and connect with others' emotions, leading to stronger and more meaningful relationships.

Better communication: Empathy can help us communicate more effectively by understanding others' perspectives and tailoring our responses accordingly.

Enhanced well-being: Empathy can lead to greater feelings of happiness, satisfaction, and overall well-being.

In summary, empathy is a critical component of emotional intelligence that involves understanding and connecting with others' emotions. Strategies for developing empathy skills can include listening actively, practicing perspective-taking, showing compassion, and cultivating self-awareness. Developing empathy skills can lead to numerous benefits, including improved relationships, better communication, and enhanced well-being.

Chapter 11:
Social Skills: Managing Others' Emotions

In this chapter, we will explore the fifth and final component of emotional intelligence - social skills - and how to develop our ability to manage others' emotions.

The Importance of Social Skills

Social skills are the ability to effectively manage and

influence the emotions of others. They are a crucial component of successful relationships and leadership. Developing social skills can help us build strong and positive relationships with others, navigate conflicts, and lead effectively.

Strategies for Developing Social Skills

There are several strategies you can use to develop social skills, including:

Communicating effectively:

Communicating clearly and effectively can help you manage others' emotions by avoiding misunderstandings and conflicts.

Building rapport:
Building rapport with others by showing interest in their experiences and perspectives can help you connect with them on a deeper level and manage their emotions more effectively.

Assertiveness: Being assertive can help you manage others' emotions by setting clear boundaries and expectations.

Active listening:

Listening actively to others' perspectives and emotions can help you manage their emotions more effectively.

The Benefits of Social Skills

Developing social skills can have numerous benefits, including:

Improved relationships:

Social skills can help us build strong and positive relationships with others, leading to greater trust and connection.

Effective leadership: Social skills are essential for effective leadership, enabling leaders to manage and influence the emotions of their team members.

Conflict resolution: Social skills can help us navigate conflicts and resolve disagreements more effectively, reducing stress and improving relationships.

In summary, social skills are the ability to effectively manage and influence the emotions of others. Strategies for developing social skills can include communicating effectively, building rapport, being assertive, and active listening. Developing social skills can lead to numerous benefits, including improved relationships, effective leadership, and conflict resolution.

Part 3: Cultivating Positive Emotions

Chapter 12:
The Benefits of Positive Emotions

In this chapter, we will explore the importance and benefits of positive emotions and how we can cultivate them in our lives.

The Power of Positive Emotions

Positive emotions are emotions that make us feel good, such as joy, gratitude, contentment, and love. These emotions have been shown to have numerous benefits for our mental and physical health, including:

Improved well-being: Positive emotions are associated with greater levels of happiness, life satisfaction, and overall well-being.

Reduced stress: Positive emotions can help us cope with stress and adversity more effectively.

Improved physical health: Positive emotions have been linked to lower levels of inflammation, improved cardiovascular health, and a stronger immune system.

Improved relationships: Positive emotions can enhance our social connections and relationships with others.

Strategies for Cultivating Positive Emotions

There are several strategies we can use to cultivate positive emotions in our lives, including:

Gratitude: Practicing gratitude by focusing on the things we are thankful for can help us cultivate positive emotions such as joy and contentment.

Mindfulness: Being present and mindful can help us appreciate the positive moments in our lives and cultivate positive emotions.

Positive self-talk: Using positive self-talk and reframing negative thoughts can help us shift our focus toward positive emotions.

Engaging in enjoyable activities: Engaging in activities we enjoy and that bring us pleasure can help us cultivate positive emotions.

The Importance of Balance

While positive emotions are important, it's also important to maintain balance and acknowledge and address negative emotions when they arise. Suppressing or ignoring negative emotions can lead to negative consequences, such as increased stress and anxiety.

In summary, positive emotions have numerous benefits for our mental and physical health, including improved well-being, reduced stress, improved physical health, and improved relationships. Strategies for cultivating positive emotions can include gratitude, mindfulness, positive self-talk, and engaging in enjoyable activities. It's important to maintain balance and acknowledge negative emotions as well.

Chapter 13:
Gratitude: Appreciating What You Have

In this chapter, we will explore the importance of gratitude and how to cultivate gratitude practice in our lives.

The Power of Gratitude

Gratitude is the practice of focusing on the things we are thankful for, both big and small. Practicing gratitude has been shown to have numerous benefits for our mental and physical health, including:

Improved well-being: Gratitude is associated with greater levels of happiness, life satisfaction, and overall well-being.

Reduced stress: Gratitude can help us cope with stress and adversity more effectively.

Improved relationships: Gratitude can enhance our social connections and relationships with others.

Improved physical health: Gratitude has been linked to lower levels of inflammation, improved cardiovascular health, and a stronger immune system.

Strategies for Cultivating Gratitude

There are several strategies we can use to cultivate a gratitude practice in our lives, including:

Gratitude journaling:

Writing down things we are grateful for each day can help us focus on the positive aspects of our lives.

Gratitude meditation:

Meditating on things we are grateful for can help us cultivate a sense of gratitude and appreciation.

Gratitude letters: Writing letters expressing gratitude to people we appreciate can help us deepen our relationships and enhance our sense of gratitude.

Gratitude walks: Going for a walk and focusing on the things we are grateful for in nature or our surroundings can help us cultivate a sense of gratitude.

Incorporating Gratitude into Daily Life

Incorporating gratitude into our daily lives can help us cultivate a more positive and appreciative mindset. Some ways to do this include:

Starting the day with gratitude: Taking a few minutes each morning to focus on things we are grateful for can set a positive tone for the day.

Practicing gratitude during daily activities: Focusing on the positive aspects of our daily activities, such as enjoying a meal or spending time with loved ones, can help us cultivate gratitude.

Expressing gratitude to others: Expressing gratitude to others for their kindness or support can help us deepen our relationships and enhance our sense of gratitude.

In summary, practicing gratitude can have numerous benefits for our mental and physical health, including improved well-being, reduced stress, improved relationships, and improved physical health. Strategies for cultivating gratitude can include gratitude journaling, meditation, letters, and walks. Incorporating gratitude into daily life can help us cultivate a more positive and appreciative mindset.

Chapter 14:
Joy: Finding Pleasure in Life

In this chapter, we will explore the importance of joy and how to cultivate joy in our lives.

What is Joy?

Joy is a feeling of pleasure or happiness that comes from experiencing something positive or meaningful. Joy can be experienced in many ways, such as through social interactions, physical activities, creative pursuits, or spiritual practices. Joy is an important part of a fulfilling life, as it can enhance our overall well-being and sense of happiness.

The Benefits of Joy

Experiencing joy can have numerous benefits for our mental and physical health, including:

Increased happiness: Joy can enhance our sense of happiness and overall well-being.

Reduced stress: Joy can help us cope with stress and adversity more effectively.

Improved relationships: Joy can enhance our social connections and relationships with others.

Improved physical health: Joy has been linked to lower levels of inflammation, improved cardiovascular health, and a stronger immune system.

Strategies for Cultivating Joy

There are several strategies we can use to cultivate joy in our lives, including:

Doing things we enjoy: Engaging in activities we find enjoyable or meaningful can help us experience joy.

Cultivating positive relationships: Spending time with people we enjoy being around and who support us can enhance our sense of joy.

Practicing mindfulness: Being present at the moment and savoring positive experiences can help us cultivate joy.

Cultivating gratitude: Focusing on the positive

aspects of our lives and feeling grateful for them can enhance our overall sense of joy.

Overcoming Barriers to Joy

Sometimes we may experience barriers to experiencing joy, such as stress, negative thoughts, or difficult life circumstances. In these cases, it can be helpful to:

Practice self-care: Taking care of our physical and

emotional needs can help us reduce stress and enhance our ability to experience joy.

Reframe negative thoughts: Reframing negative thoughts into more positive or constructive ones can help us shift our mindset and enhance our ability to experience joy.

Seek support: Reaching out to others for support and guidance can help us overcome barriers to experiencing joy.

In summary, joy is an important part of a fulfilling life and can enhance our overall well-being and sense of happiness. Strategies for cultivating joy can include doing things we enjoy, cultivating positive relationships, practicing mindfulness, and cultivating gratitude. Overcoming barriers to joy may involve practicing self-care, reframing negative

thoughts, and seeking
support.

Chapter 15:
Love: Connecting with Others

In this chapter, we will explore the importance of love in our lives and how to cultivate love in our relationships with others.

What is Love?

Love is a complex emotion that can take many forms, such as romantic love, familial love, or platonic love. Love involves feelings of warmth, caring, and compassion toward others, and it can enhance our sense of connection and belonging.

The Benefits of Love

Experiencing love can have numerous benefits for our mental and physical health, including:

Increased happiness: Love can enhance our sense of

happiness and overall well-being.

Reduced stress: Love can help us cope with stress and adversity more effectively.

Improved relationships: Love can enhance our social connections and relationships with others.

Improved physical health: Love has been linked to lower levels of inflammation, improved cardiovascular health, and a stronger immune system.

Strategies for Cultivating Love

There are several strategies we can use to cultivate love in our relationships with others, including:

Practicing kindness: Showing kindness and compassion toward others can help cultivate feelings of love and connection.

Communicating effectively: Communicating openly and

honestly with others can enhance our ability to connect and feel loved.

Practicing empathy: Seeking to understand others' perspectives and experiences can enhance our ability to connect and feel loved.

Cultivating gratitude: Focusing on the positive aspects of our relationships and feeling grateful for them can enhance our overall sense of love.

Overcoming Barriers to Love

Sometimes we may experience barriers to experiencing love, such as past traumas, negative relationship patterns, or difficult life circumstances. In these cases, it can be helpful to:

Seek therapy: Working with a therapist can help us address past traumas and negative relationship patterns that may be preventing us from experiencing love.

Practice self-compassion: Being kind and compassionate toward ourselves can help us overcome self-doubt or negative self-talk that may be preventing us from experiencing love.

Practice forgiveness: Forgiving others for past hurts can help us move past resentments and cultivate feelings of love and compassion.

In summary, love is an important emotion that can enhance our sense of connection and belonging. Strategies for cultivating love can include practicing kindness, communicating effectively, practicing empathy, and cultivating gratitude. Overcoming barriers to love may involve seeking therapy, practicing self-compassion, and practicing forgiveness.

Chapter 16:
Hope: Looking Toward the Future

In this chapter, we will explore the importance of hope in our lives and how to cultivate hope even in difficult circumstances.

What is Hope?

Hope is an emotion that involves a positive expectation about the future, even in the face of adversity or uncertainty. It involves a belief that things will improve, and that we have the ability to influence positive outcomes.

The Benefits of Hope

Experiencing hope can have numerous benefits for our mental and physical health, including:

Improved well-being: Hope can enhance our sense of optimism and overall well-being.

Increased resilience: Hope can help us cope with difficult situations and rebound from setbacks more easily.

Improved relationships: Hope can enhance our social connections and relationships with others.

Improved physical health: Hope has been linked to improved immune function, lower rates of chronic illness, and faster recovery from illness or injury.

Strategies for Cultivating Hope

There are several strategies we can use to cultivate hope, even in difficult circumstances, including:

Setting realistic goals: Setting achievable goals and working toward them can help us build a sense of optimism and hope for the future.

Focusing on strengths: Identifying and utilizing our strengths can help us build confidence in our ability to influence positive outcomes.

Seeking support: Connecting with supportive friends, family members, or a therapist can help us maintain a positive outlook and build resilience in the face of adversity.

Practicing gratitude: Focusing on the positive

aspects of our lives and feeling grateful for them can help us maintain a sense of hope, even in difficult times.

Overcoming Barriers to Hope

Sometimes we may experience barriers to experiencing hope, such as chronic illness, loss, or trauma. In these cases, it can be helpful to:

Seek support: Connecting with others who have

experienced similar challenges can help us build a sense of hope and resilience.

Focus on small steps: Breaking down large goals into smaller, achievable steps can help us maintain a sense of progress and hope.

Practice self-compassion: Being kind and compassionate toward ourselves can help us maintain a positive outlook, even in difficult circumstances.

In summary, hope is an important emotion that can enhance our sense of optimism, resilience, and overall well-being. Strategies for cultivating hope can include setting realistic goals, focusing on strengths, seeking support, and practicing gratitude. Overcoming barriers to hope may involve seeking support, focusing on small steps, and practicing self-compassion.

Chapter 17:
Forgiveness: Letting Go of Negative Emotions

In this chapter, we will explore the concept of forgiveness and its importance in managing negative emotions.

What is Forgiveness?

Forgiveness is the act of letting go of anger, resentment, or negative feelings toward someone who has wronged us. It involves choosing to release the negative emotions associated with a particular event or person and can be a powerful tool for managing our own emotional well-being.

The Benefits of Forgiveness

Forgiveness can have numerous benefits for our mental and physical health, including:

Reduced stress and anxiety: Holding onto anger and resentment can contribute to stress and anxiety, while forgiveness can help us feel more calm and relaxed.

Improved relationships: Forgiveness can help repair damaged relationships and enhance our social connections with others.

Increased empathy: Forgiveness can help us develop greater empathy and understanding for others, even those who have wronged us.

Improved mental health: Forgiveness has been linked to lower rates of depression and anxiety, and can improve our overall mental health and well-being.

Strategies for Practicing Forgiveness

Practicing forgiveness can be challenging, but there are several strategies that can help us let go of negative emotions and cultivate forgiveness, including:

Acknowledge the hurt: Recognizing the pain and hurt caused by someone's actions can help us begin to process our emotions and move toward forgiveness.

Practice empathy: Trying to understand the perspective of the person who wronged us can help us develop greater empathy and compassion.

Consider the benefits of forgiveness: Reflecting on the potential benefits of forgiveness, such as improved relationships and reduced stress, can help motivate us to let go of negative emotions.

Take small steps: Forgiveness is a process, and it may take time to fully release negative emotions. Taking small steps, such as practicing empathy or focusing on the present moment, can help us move toward forgiveness over time.

Overcoming Barriers to Forgiveness

Sometimes, we may experience barriers to practicing forgiveness, such as feelings of anger, hurt, or fear. In these cases, it can be helpful to:

Seek support: Connecting with supportive friends or a therapist can help us process our emotions and work toward forgiveness.

Practice self-compassion: Being kind and compassionate toward ourselves can help us release negative emotions and cultivate forgiveness.

Practice mindfulness: Focusing on the present

moment and cultivating a sense of mindfulness can help us let go of negative emotions and move toward forgiveness.

In summary, forgiveness is a powerful tool for managing negative emotions and improving our mental and physical health. Strategies for practicing forgiveness can include acknowledging the hurt, practicing empathy, considering the benefits, and taking small steps. Overcoming barriers to forgiveness may involve seeking support, practicing self-compassion, and cultivating mindfulness.

Part 4: Overcoming Negative Emotions

Chapter 18:
The Impact of Negative Emotions

In this chapter, we will explore the impact of negative emotions on our mental and physical health.

What Are Negative Emotions?

Negative emotions are feelings such as anger, sadness, fear, and anxiety that can have a detrimental impact on our well-being. These emotions can be triggered by various events, such as conflict with others, difficult life transitions, or traumatic experiences.

The Effects of Negative Emotions

Negative emotions can have a range of effects on our mental and physical health, including:

Increased stress: Negative emotions can trigger the body's stress response, leading to physical symptoms such as increased heart rate, muscle tension, and shallow breathing.

Decreased immune function: Chronic negative emotions can weaken the immune system, making us more vulnerable to illness and disease.

Increased risk of mental health disorders: Prolonged negative emotions can increase the risk of mental health disorders such as depression and anxiety.

Impaired relationships: Negative emotions can strain relationships with others, leading to conflict and communication difficulties.

Reduced quality of life: Chronic negative emotions can reduce our overall quality of life and contribute to feelings of unhappiness and dissatisfaction.

Strategies for Managing Negative Emotions

While negative emotions can be challenging to manage, there are several strategies that can help us cope with these feelings, including:

Mindfulness: Practicing mindfulness can help us become more aware of our negative emotions and develop a more accepting and non-judgmental attitude toward them.

Cognitive restructuring: Changing our negative thought patterns and beliefs can help us reframe our emotions and feel more positive and optimistic.

Emotional regulation: Learning to regulate our emotions through techniques such as deep breathing, progressive muscle relaxation, or meditation can help us manage intense negative feelings.

Seeking support: Connecting with supportive friends, family, or a therapist can help us process our negative emotions and work through difficult feelings.

Developing Resilience to Negative Emotions

In addition to managing negative emotions, developing resilience can help us cope with challenging situations and experiences. Strategies for building resilience can include:

Cultivating a sense of purpose and meaning in life

Building strong social connections

Practicing self-care and self-compassion

Fostering optimism and a positive outlook

In summary, negative emotions can have a significant impact on our mental and physical health. Strategies for managing negative emotions can include mindfulness, cognitive restructuring, emotional regulation, and seeking support. Developing resilience can also help us cope with difficult emotions and experiences.

Chapter 19:
Anger: Understanding and Managing It

Anger is a powerful emotion that can have both positive and negative effects on our lives. In this chapter, we will explore the causes and consequences of anger, as well as strategies for managing this emotion effectively.

What Is Anger?

Anger is an emotional response to a perceived threat or injustice. It is a natural and normal emotion that everyone experiences at times, but it can become problematic when it is expressed inappropriately or excessively.

Causes of Anger

Anger can be caused by a variety of factors, including:

Frustration with a situation or person

Feeling threatened or attacked

Feeling powerless or out of control

Feeling disrespected or mistreated

Consequences of Anger

While anger can sometimes be a useful emotion, it can also have negative consequences, including:

Damaged relationships: Anger can cause us to lash out at others, damaging our relationships and creating conflict.

Health problems: Prolonged anger can lead to health problems such as high blood pressure and heart disease.

Legal issues: Uncontrolled anger can lead to legal issues such as assault or domestic violence.

Negative self-image: Chronic anger can damage our self-image and lead to feelings of shame or guilt.

Strategies for Managing Anger

While it can be challenging to manage anger, there are several strategies that can help us control this emotion, including:

Identify triggers: Becoming aware of the situations or people that trigger our anger can help us prepare and respond in a more constructive way.

Practice relaxation techniques: Techniques such as deep breathing, meditation, and yoga can help us manage our physical responses to anger.

Reframe negative thoughts: Learning to reframe negative thoughts can help us respond to situations in a more positive and constructive way.

Seek support: Talking to a trusted friend, family member, or therapist can provide a supportive outlet for our anger.

Seeking Professional Help

If anger is causing significant problems in our lives, it may be helpful to seek professional help from a therapist or counselor. Therapy can help us explore the underlying causes of our anger and develop more effective strategies for managing this emotion.

In summary, anger is a powerful emotion that can have both positive and negative effects on our lives. By understanding the causes and consequences of anger and developing effective strategies for managing this emotion, we can improve our relationships and overall well-being.

Chapter 20:
Fear: Confronting Your Anxieties

Fear is a common and natural emotion that arises in response to perceived danger or threat. While fear can be helpful in certain situations, it can also become overwhelming and limit our ability to live our lives to the fullest. In this chapter, we will explore the nature of fear, the ways in which it can impact our lives, and strategies for confronting our anxieties.

What Is Fear?

Fear is an emotion that is triggered by a perceived threat to our physical or emotional well-being. It is a survival mechanism that helps us respond to danger by triggering the fight-or-flight response.

Types of Fear

There are many types of fear, including:

Phobias: Intense and irrational fears of specific objects or situations.

Panic disorder: Sudden and intense feelings of fear that can be triggered by specific situations or events.

Generalized anxiety disorder: A chronic and

excessive worry about many different things.

Consequences of Fear

While fear can sometimes be helpful, it can also have negative consequences, including:

Avoidance behavior: Fear can cause us to avoid situations or activities that we perceive as threatening, limiting our experiences and opportunities.

Physical symptoms: Fear can cause physical symptoms such as sweating, rapid heartbeat, and trembling, which can be uncomfortable and distressing.

Negative self-talk: Fear can lead to negative self-talk, which can damage our self-esteem and create a negative cycle of anxiety.

Strategies for Confronting Fear

There are several strategies that can help us confront our fears and manage our anxiety, including:

Exposure therapy: Gradually exposing ourselves to the source of our fear in a safe and controlled environment can help us desensitize to it over time.

Mindfulness: Practicing mindfulness can help us become more aware of our thoughts and emotions and learn to respond to them in a more constructive way.

Cognitive-behavioral therapy: This type of therapy can help us identify and reframe negative thoughts and beliefs that contributed to our anxiety.

Self-care: Engaging in activities that promote self-care, such as exercise, meditation, and spending time with loved ones, can help us reduce our stress levels and manage our anxiety.

Seeking Professional Help

If fear is significantly impacting our ability to function in our daily lives, it may be helpful to seek professional help from a therapist or counselor.

Therapy can provide us with the tools and support we need to confront our fears and manage our anxiety.

In conclusion, fear is a natural and sometimes helpful emotion, but it can also become overwhelming and limit our ability to live our lives to the fullest. By understanding the nature of fear, recognizing its impact on our lives, and using effective strategies for confronting our anxieties, we can learn to manage our anxiety and live more fulfilling lives.

Chapter 21:
Sadness: Coping with Loss and Grief

Sadness is a natural emotion that we all experience at some point in our lives. It can arise from various situations, such as the loss of a loved one, a breakup, or even a disappointment. While it's normal to feel sad from time to time, prolonged sadness or grief can be debilitating and even lead to depression.

In this chapter, we'll explore the different causes of sadness and grief, and how to cope with them. We'll discuss the stages of grief and the different coping mechanisms that can help us deal with the loss of a loved one. We'll also talk about the importance of self-care during this time and how to build a support system to help us through the grieving process.

Additionally, we'll discuss the difference between sadness and depression and when to seek professional help. We'll look at how to recognize the signs of depression and how to take the first steps toward seeking help. Finally, we'll explore the different treatments available for depression, including different therapies.

The difference between sadness and depression.

Sadness and depression are both emotional states, but they differ in intensity and duration. Sadness is a feeling of unhappiness or disappointment that is usually temporary and milder than depression. Sadness is often caused by a loss or disappointment, while depression is often more persistent and intense. Depression is an umbrella term used to describe a range of mental health disorders, such as major depressive disorder and dysthymia.

When sadness becomes prolonged and difficult to manage, it may be time to seek professional help. If you find yourself crying more than usual, feeling hopeless or worthless, having difficulty concentrating, or having difficulty performing day-to-day activities, it may be a sign of depression and you should seek help from a mental health professional. Professional help can provide you with strategies and resources to manage your symptoms and provide support as you work through your feelings.

How to recognize the signs of depression and how to take steps toward seeking help.

1. Recognizing the Signs of Depression:

- Persistent sad, anxious, or "empty" mood

- Loss of interest or pleasure in activities that were once enjoyed

- Feelings of guilt, worthlessness, helplessness, and/or hopelessness

- Fatigue and decreased energy

- Difficulty concentrating, remembering details, and making decisions

- Insomnia, early-morning wakefulness, or excessive sleeping

- Appetite and/or weight changes

- Thoughts of death or suicide, or suicide attempts

- Aches and pains, headaches, cramps, or digestive problems without a clear physical cause

2. Taking steps toward Seeking Help:

- Talk to someone you trust, such as a friend, family

member, or health professional.

- Reach out to a support group or counseling service.

- Find an online forum or support group.

- Seek help from your religious or spiritual group.

- Research mental health services in your area.

- Make an appointment with a mental health professional.

Therapy treatments: **Cognitive Behavioral Therapy (CBT)**

Cognitive Behavioral Therapy (CBT) is a type of psychotherapy that focuses on changing negative thought patterns and behaviors. It is based on the belief that our thoughts, feelings, and behaviors are all connected, and that by changing one, we can influence the others. CBT can help people learn to recognize and manage their own thoughts and feelings, as well as learn new, more adaptive behaviors.

CBT works by helping people identify and challenge their negative thoughts and beliefs. This process helps people become aware of how their thoughts affect their feelings and behaviors, and how they can take steps to challenge the negative thoughts. Once the negative thoughts are challenged, people can then start to focus on more positive thoughts and behaviors.

CBT focuses on the present, rather than the past. It also emphasizes problem-solving and action. Through this approach, people learn to identify their triggers and develop coping strategies so they can better manage their negative thoughts and behaviors.

CBT can be used to treat a wide range of issues, including anxiety, depression, post-traumatic stress disorder, relationships, substance abuse, eating disorders, and more. It is also often used in combination with other therapies, such as medication, lifestyle changes, and self-care.

Interpersonal Therapy

Interpersonal therapy (IPT) is an evidence-based, time-limited form of psychotherapy that focuses on how current relationships, including those with family and friends, contribute to a person's mental health. IPT helps people to develop better communication and problem-solving skills, and to improve their overall relationships with others. It can be used to treat a variety of mental health conditions, such as depression, anxiety, eating disorders, and substance abuse.

The goal of IPT is to help people identify and understand their current interpersonal difficulties and develop strategies to better manage them. During IPT, the therapist helps the client to recognize patterns in his or her relationships, identify and modify unhelpful behaviors, and develop better communication and problem-solving skills. They may also focus on the client's goals for the future and how to achieve them.

IPT typically consists of 12 to 16 weekly sessions, with each session lasting 45-50 minutes. During the first few sessions, the therapist will explore the client's current interpersonal issues and past relationships. The therapist will then work with the client to help them identify any unhelpful behaviors that may be contributing to the problem.

Throughout the course of treatment, the therapist will continue to provide support and help the client work on developing better communication and problem-solving skills. The therapist may also provide guidance and support in identifying and making changes in the client's relationships with family and friends.

Dialectical Behavioral Therapy (DBT)

Dialectical Behavioral Therapy (DBT) is a type of cognitive-behavioral therapy that focuses on helping people develop skills to manage their emotions, thoughts, and behaviors. This type of therapy is rooted in the concept of dialectics, which is the idea that opposing forces can both be true. In DBT, the therapist and client work together to understand both sides of a situation and to find a way to move forward. DBT is used to help people cope with challenging situations, such as addiction, depression, and relationship issues. DBT focuses on teaching clients some vital skills like mindfulness, distress tolerance, emotion regulation, and interpersonal effectiveness, which are meant to help people better regulate their emotions, better manage their relationships and conflicts, and develop healthier, more fulfilling lives.

Below are explanations of some of the skills:
 Mindfulness:

Mindfulness is the practice of being aware and present in the moment. With DBT, mindfulness can help you become more aware of your emotions and understand them better. Regularly practice mindfulness exercises such as deep breathing, meditation, and focusing on the present moment.

Distress Tolerance Therapy: DBT teaches skills to help you manage and cope with distress. Try to practice distraction techniques such as taking a walk, listening to music, or engaging in a hobby when feeling overwhelmed.

Emotion Regulation: Emotion regulation skills help you manage and regulate your emotions in a healthy way. Practice self-soothing techniques such as journaling, deep breathing, and positive self-talk.

Interpersonal Effectiveness: Interpersonal effectiveness skills help you to effectively communicate in relationships. Practice effective communication techniques such as active listening, speaking assertively, and understanding body language.

Recognize and Label Emotions: It is important to be able to identify and label your emotions in order to better understand and manage them. Try to practice recognizing and labeling your feelings throughout the day.

Acceptance and Commitment Therapy (ACT)

Acceptance and Commitment Therapy (ACT) is an evidence-based psychological intervention that helps individuals build psychological flexibility and live a meaningful life in the presence of difficult thoughts and feelings. ACT teaches people how to observe their experience without judging or trying to change it. This helps to reduce stress and improve emotional well-being.

 ACT helps people to identify personal values and create goals based on them. This allows individuals to live in line with their values and move towards a meaningful life.

ACT encourages people to take committed action toward their goals. This helps people to break free from patterns of avoidance and inaction that can lead to feelings of helplessness.

ACT helps individuals to develop mindfulness skills to improve their ability to be present in the moment. This helps people to be more aware of their choices and take action that is consistent with their values.

ACT teaches individuals to become more aware of their thinking patterns and how they can influence their behavior. This helps people to identify unhelpful thinking patterns and replace them with more helpful ones.

ACT helps individuals to develop perspective-taking skills to gain insight into the impact their thoughts and behaviors have on others. This helps people to become more compassionate and understanding of themselves and others.

Eye Movement Desensitization and Reprocessing (EMDR)

Eye Movement Desensitization and Reprocessing (EMDR) is an evidence-based psychotherapy treatment that was developed by Francine Shapiro in the late 1980s.

 It is based on the idea that when a person is exposed to a traumatic or distressing event, their natural coping mechanisms become overwhelmed and the memory of the event becomes "stuck" in the brain. EMDR aims to help the individual reprocess memories by stimulating the brain with eye movements. Eye movements are thought to help the brain to access memories and process them in a more adaptive way.

During EMDR, the therapist will ask the client to recall their traumatic memory while focusing on a back-and-forth movement of the eyes. The client is then asked to report on their experience. The therapist will then offer the client cognitive, emotional, and physical interventions to help them process their traumatic memories more effectively. EMDR can be used to treat many conditions, including post-traumatic stress disorder (PTSD), depression, anxiety, and phobias.

Clinical research has found that EMDR is effective in reducing symptoms of trauma, and many individuals report feeling significantly better after just a few sessions.

Mindfulness-Based Cognitive Therapy (MBCT)

MBCT is an evidence-based psychological therapy that combines elements of mindfulness meditation and cognitive behavioral therapy (CBT) to help people manage their depression, anxiety, and other mental health issues. MBCT teaches individuals to recognize and modify negative thought patterns and behaviors, increase awareness of one's emotions, and learn to live in the present moment. Through this combination of cognitive and mindfulness-based techniques, MBCT helps individuals become more aware of their thoughts and feelings and, in turn, develop healthier ways of responding to their distress.

Some of the key components of MBCT include:

• Learning to recognize and challenge negative thoughts and beliefs.

• Practicing mindfulness by focusing on the present moment rather than dwelling on the past or worrying about the future

• Developing self-compassion and self-acceptance

• Identifying and changing patterns of avoidance

• Developing healthier behaviors and strategies for managing difficult emotions

• Applying mindfulness to everyday activities

• Learning to recognize and accept difficult emotions without judging them.

MBCT can be beneficial for people who have experienced depression, anxiety, stress, and other mental health issues. It can also help those who are struggling with chronic pain or other physical health conditions.

Family Therapy

• Family therapy can be used to help families form healthier relationships by improving communication and resolving conflicts.

• Family therapy can help family members better understand each other's feelings and perspectives, and to develop healthier ways of expressing and resolving conflicts.

• Family therapy can help family members learn to recognize and express emotion in healthy ways.

• Family therapy can help family members learn to identify and manage stress, and to build positive relationships within the family.

• Family therapy can help family members develop

problem-solving skills, which can be used to find solutions to challenging family issues.

•	Family therapy can help family members develop better-coping skills and create a more positive family environment.

•	Family therapy can help family members learn to recognize and accept individual differences, and to develop a sense of empathy and understanding.

- Family therapy can help family members learn to make better decisions for their family as a whole.

- Family therapy can help family members recognize and manage feelings of anger, sadness, fear, and other emotions in a healthy way.

- Family therapy can help family members learn to appreciate each other and foster healthy relationships.

For Medical Treatments for depression, working with a healthcare provider or mental health professional is advised. It's better to collaborate with a healthcare physician or mental health expert to create a plan that is specific to your requirements

Chapter 22:
Guilt and Shame: Letting Go of Regret

Guilt and shame are powerful emotions that can have a profound impact on our mental health and well-being. While guilt can be a useful emotion that helps us recognize when we've done something wrong, it can also be overwhelming and lead to feelings of shame and self-blame. Shame, on the other hand, is a more complex emotion that involves feeling unworthy or defective as a person.

In this chapter, we'll explore the causes and effects of guilt and shame, and how to let go of regret. We'll discuss the difference between healthy guilt and toxic guilt, and how to manage feelings of shame and self-blame.

By the end of this chapter, you'll have a better

understanding of guilt and shame and how to let go of regret. You'll be able to recognize when guilt or shame is becoming overwhelming and have tools to manage those feelings. You'll also have a better understanding of the role of self-forgiveness and self-compassion in healing from guilt and shame.

Causes of Guilt and Shame

1. Feeling responsible for a negative event or outcome.

2. Engaging in an immoral or unethical behavior.

3. Blaming yourself for something that is out of your control.

4. Not meeting your own standards or expectations.

5. Taking on other people's feelings or experiences.

Effects of Guilt and Shame

1. Low self-esteem and self-worth.

2. Isolation and withdrawal from social situations.

3. Self-destructive behaviors such as substance abuse.

4. Depression and anxiety.

5. Difficulty making decisions or taking action.

Letting Go of Regret

1. Acknowledge your feelings of guilt and shame and accept that they are valid.

2. Talk to someone you trust or seek professional help if needed.

3. Let go of the need to control the outcome and practice self-compassion.

4. Identify the lessons learned and focus on the positive.

5. Make amends if necessary and forgive yourself.

The difference between healthy guilt and toxic guilt.

Healthy guilt and toxic guilt are two different forms of guilt that have different effects on our mental health. Healthy guilt is a normal emotion that motivates us to correct our mistakes or take responsibility for our actions. It can be a useful tool for self-reflection and improvement. On the other hand, toxic guilt is a debilitating emotion that can lead to feelings of shame and self-blame. It often stems from unrealistic expectations or false beliefs, and it can cause us to feel overwhelmed and unable to make decisions.

The best way to manage feelings of shame and self-blame is to practice self-compassion.

Self-compassion involves being kind and understanding towards yourself, accepting your mistakes and shortcomings, and recognizing that everyone makes mistakes. It is important to recognize that you are not your mistakes and to forgive yourself.

Additionally, it can be helpful to challenge any negative self-talk and to reframe your mistakes as opportunities for growth and learning. Lastly, it can be beneficial to practice mindfulness and to focus on the present moment instead of ruminating on the past or worrying about the future.

Overall, it is important to recognize the difference between healthy and toxic guilt and to engage in self-care practices to manage feelings of shame and self-blame. Practicing self-compassion, challenging negative self-talk, and focusing on the present are all helpful strategies for managing guilt and shame.

Chapter 23:
Stress: Managing the Demands of Life

Stress is an unavoidable part of life, and it can have a significant impact on our emotional and physical well-being. In this chapter, we'll explore the causes and effects of stress, and how to manage it effectively.

We'll begin by discussing the different types of stress

and how they impact our bodies and minds. Several factors contribute to stress, such as work, relationships, and financial pressures. Also, some of the physical symptoms of stress, include headaches, muscle tension, and insomnia.

We'll then delve into different stress management techniques, such as deep breathing, and exercise. Furthermore, we'll examine the role of positive thinking and reframing negative thoughts in managing stress. We'll also explore how to set realistic goals and expectations and manage time effectively to reduce stress levels.

Finally, we'll discuss the importance of seeking help when stress becomes overwhelming and how to find support from family, friends, and professionals.

By the end of this chapter, you'll have a better

understanding of stress and how to manage it effectively. You'll have tools and techniques to reduce stress levels and prioritize self-care, and you'll know how to seek help when stress becomes too much to handle.

Causes of Stress:

1. Financial Problems: Struggling to make ends meet or worrying about the

future can cause a great deal of stress.

2. Work: High-pressure work environments, long hours, and an unclear future can cause stress.

3. Unhealthy Lifestyle: Poor diet, lack of sleep, and lack of exercise can all lead to stress.

4. Family Difficulties: Family arguments and disagreements can be a major source of stress.

5. Relationship Issues: Struggling to maintain a healthy relationship can be stressful.

6. Health Problems: Chronic or serious health issues can cause a great deal of stress.

Effects of Stress:

1. Physical: Stress can lead to physical problems such as headaches, stomachaches, and fatigue.

2. Mental: Stress can lead to anxiety, depression, and irritability.

3. Emotional: Stress can lead to feelings of sadness, helplessness, and fear.

How to Manage Stress Effectively:

1. Exercise: Regular physical activity can help to reduce stress levels.

2. Talk to Someone: Talking to a friend, family member,

or professional can help to relieve stress.

3. Get Enough Sleep: A lack of sleep can increase stress levels, so getting enough rest is important.

4. Manage Time: Learning how to better manage your time can help to reduce stress.

5. Take Breaks: Taking breaks throughout the day can help to reduce stress levels.

6. Practice Relaxation Techniques: Techniques such as deep breathing, yoga, and meditation can help to reduce stress.

The different types of stress and how they impact our bodies and minds
1. Physical Stress: Physical stress is caused by physical exertion, injury, or illness. It can cause a variety of symptoms, such as fatigue, pain, muscle tension, headaches, and digestive

problems. It can also lead to sleep disturbances, anxiety, and depression.

2. Emotional Stress: Emotional stress is caused by difficult life events, such as relationship problems, job loss, financial strain, or the death of a loved one. It can lead to physical symptoms, such as headaches, chest pain, and an increased heart rate. It can also cause changes in behavior, mood, and attitude.

3. Mental Stress: Mental stress is caused by worrying

or feeling overwhelmed. It can lead to anxiety, depression, and other mental health issues. It can also cause physical symptoms, such as insomnia, fatigue, and muscle tension.

4. Social Stress: Social stress is caused by social situations, such as work, school, or family conflict. It can lead to physical symptoms, such as

headaches, stomachaches, and nausea. It can also affect your mood and attitude.

5. Environmental Stress: Environmental stress is caused by environmental factors, such as extreme temperatures, noise, or pollution. It can lead to physical symptoms, such as fatigue, headaches, and digestive problems. It can also affect your mood and your ability to concentrate.

1. Deep Breathing: Deep breathing is a simple and effective stress management technique that can be done anywhere and anytime. It helps reduce tension and anxiety while calming your mind. To get started, find a comfortable spot, close your eyes and take a few slow, deep breaths in through your nose and out through your mouth. Focus on the feeling of the air going in and out of your body. This

practice can help to reset your mental and physical state.

2. Exercise: Exercise is an excellent way to reduce stress and improve your overall wellbeing. Regular physical activity can help to improve mood and reduce feelings of tension or anxiety. It can also help to reduce the production of stress hormones. Find an activity you enjoy, such as walking, running, swimming or cycling, and aim to do it for at least 30 minutes a few times a week.

3. Meditation: Meditation is a powerful stress management technique that can help to clear your mind and reduce stress levels. Find a comfortable spot, close your eyes and focus on your breathing. Pay attention to how your body feels and the sensations you experience. This practice can help to quiet your thoughts and create a sense of peace and balance.

4. Positive Self-Talk: Negative self-talk can cause and exacerbate stress. Try to replace negative thoughts with positive ones. Speak to yourself as you would a friend in need and focus on the things you are grateful for.

5. Get Outdoors: The outdoors can be a great stress reliever. Nature has a calming effect on the mind and the sounds, smells and sights can help to reduce feelings of stress and

anxiety. Take a walk in the park, sit in your garden or visit a local park. All of these activities can help to reduce stress.

The role of positive thinking and reframing negative thoughts in managing stress.

1 By focusing on the positives and reframing negative thoughts, we can help to gain a more balanced outlook on life and find ways to cope with stress.

2. Reframing negative thoughts can allow us to gain a better perspective on

stressful situations. Instead of thinking, "I can't do this", we can reframe the thought to "I can find a way to do this". This shift in thinking can help us to find solutions and develop more resilience in the face of stress.

3. Positive thinking can help us to stay focused on our goals and feel more empowered. When facing a stressful situation, we can remind ourselves of our strengths and use positive affirmations to keep our spirits up.

4. Reframing negative thoughts can also help us to

maintain a positive attitude toward ourselves and others. Instead of beating ourselves up for our mistakes, we can try to look at the situation objectively and find ways to learn and grow from it.

5. Positive thinking and reframing negative thoughts can help us to stay calm and focused in the face of stress. Instead of getting overwhelmed by the situation, we can look for creative solutions and look for ways to make the best of the situation.

Setting realistic goals and expectations and managing time effectively to reduce stress levels.

1. Identify Your Goals: Take some time to think about what you want to achieve in the short and long term. Make sure your goals are realistic and achievable.

2. Break Your Goals Down: Once you've identified your goals, break them down into smaller, more manageable tasks. This will make them

less overwhelming and more achievable.

3. Prioritize Your Tasks: Make sure to prioritize the tasks that will lead you closer to your goals. This will help you focus on what's important and give you a sense of accomplishment.

4. Set a Timetable: Create a timetable for yourself and set realistic deadlines for the tasks you need to complete. This will help you

stay organized and motivated.

5. Take Time for Yourself: Don't forget to make time for yourself. Take regular breaks, practice stress-reducing activities, and spend time with friends and family.

6. Track Your Progress: Keep track of your progress and reward yourself when you achieve your goals. This will help you stay motivated and reduce stress.

7. Ask for Help: Don't be afraid to ask for help when you need it. Talk to friends, family, or a professional if you need support or guidance.

CONCLUSION
Mastering Your Emotions for a Happier Life

In this book, we've explored the complexities of emotions and how they impact our lives. We've learned that emotions are a natural part of the human experience and play a vital role in our daily lives. We've also learned that emotions can be challenging to manage and can have a significant impact on our wellbeing.

Through exploring the science of emotions, emotional intelligence, and the benefits of positive emotions, we've gained a deeper understanding of how our emotions impact our thoughts, behaviors, and relationships.

We've also explored the impact of negative emotions, such as anger, fear, and sadness, and learned how to manage them effectively. Additionally, we've discussed stress management techniques and the importance of prioritizing self-care.

By mastering our emotions, we can lead happier, more fulfilling lives. We can develop better relationships, achieve our goals, and find greater satisfaction and meaning in our daily lives.

Remember, mastering your emotions is a lifelong journey, and it takes time, effort, and practice. However, with the tools and strategies outlined in this book, you have the foundation to take control of your emotions and lead a happier, healthier life.